The Keto Journey: Getting Past the Plateau

Jen Pitman

ISBN-13:

978-1974618439
ISBN-10:

1974618439

DEDICATION

To any person who has felt uncomfortable in their own skin. I am living proof there is life beyond your weight. Leave behind the negativity - for those words can last a lifetime. You're not alone.

TABLE OF CONTENTS

ABOUT THIS BOOK

This book is a personal, detailed report of my journey to Ketosis. If you are questioning whether this book is for you I would ask if you have ever suffered from the following thoughts. "Why can't I lose weight?", "Why have I failed diets by bingeing?", "Can I lose weight after so many years of failing?", "Can the Ketogenic Diet work for someone with a cycle of food addiction?", "Why don't other Keto books talk about the difficult personal journey I am experiencing?", or "My friends/family don't understand how hard it is for me to lose weight". All of the previous thoughts are what I struggled with for so many years. I love food! I love the chemical happiness I feel when I eat food. But, should my happiness be dependent or dictated by what I feed my body?

For more than 15 years my mind was consumed by the thought of food. What I was going to eat next, giving into irrational cravings and being excited about large quantities of food. For many, they can read all the diet books in the world that scientifically explain why a diet is beneficial. But, I want this book to be a realistic interpretation for someone who is fighting against all odds. I had become frustrated reading diet tips and tricks by individuals who stated they were always athletic as a child/teen. Individuals who only gained weight at one point in their life. Individuals who only gained fat on one part of their body.

My story never fit the books I read and I immediately felt disadvantaged by my challenges. I would push through and embark on a diet journey, following someone who has never struggled mentally and physically like I had. I would always fail. I was never an athlete, I gain weight all over my body in unison, I have cellulite in more than one 6x6 inch square on my body, I am hormonal and require high levels of estrogen, I don't enjoy working out, I stress eat, I eat when I am happy, I am genetically predisposed to love carbs and sugar, I don't have a thyroid problem that I am aware of, I have social anxiety and I was fighting my food addiction to the comfort of food. People deserve to read a true and real story of someone who is just trying to figure it all out. Let's be one another's counselor in life and share the deepest experiences so that our children and friends don't have to feel alone when they reach this crossroads. Shall we begin?

CHAPTER 1 MY STORY

My name is Jen Pitman and I am a military spouse living in Jacksonville, Florida. I had finally reached the point in my life where my body and mind were working against each other. You know the time in your life when you think "I should have listened to my mother". The long list of life changes are as follows – I lotion my body more than a newborn baby, I apply anti-wrinkle cream nightly, I scrub the dead skin from my body as suggested, I ingest earthy tasting vitamins, I wash my hair once a week (because it falls out), I abstain from tugging on the loose skin on my neck, I apply serums to my hair (because it falls out), I get my nails done routinely, I change my hair annually and those are just the cosmetic changes I have made routine in my life. You would think with all those changes I would be happy with my body but I wasn't.

I struggled with my relationship with food from early teenage years. I recall having body dysmorphia most of my life (where you see yourself fatter than you are). Puberty threw me into a tailspin of weight gain and depression. I remember coming back to high school after summer and a "rumor" had spread that I had gotten fat. If I showed you the picture of what I weighed then, you would laugh. I wasn't extremely thin but I had started getting those curves people dream of. Jealousy I suppose but I listened to the world around me and I started obsessing about my weight. I hadn't developed proper coping skills and I was fighting biology. I was depressed, gaining weight, introverted, failing in school and turning to food to feel happy. I always knew I had an eating disorder but I just didn't care. I wasn't the type to admit that I had any problem. I was "fine" for 25 years. It wasn't until I got married that I realized…Okay, admitted that I had an addiction to food. Having a partner in life exposes all of your inner demons and I could no longer make excuses for binge eating. I won't go into too much detail about my history but I will attempt to convey the feelings and emotions of having a food addiction. I'm not a doctor or a licensed professional but I am here to give you my story. Warning: some of these explanations may be triggers if you have a history of bingeing.

What do I think a food addiction is? An unhealthy, all-encompassing obsession with the thought, forethought and after thought of food and/or meals. It's a 24/7 a day job that I am not getting paid for. I vividly recall being able to turn my hunger off like a switch. I would wake up and think about food and what I was going to eat. I would dream and envision food that I could buy on my way to school or work. If I was presented with a lunch date or family gathering option I would create a back-up plan of how to eat what I wanted afterward. Living on my own also gave me free rein on what I ate, when and how much of it. Fast food was heaven. It was cheap, delicious and I could eat it at home or in my car. I would order my standard of two cheeseburgers, large fries, large coke, 10 piece nuggets and sometimes ice cream. The frantic adrenaline rush I felt was sickening. I hated every minute of needing to binge on food like I was never going to eat again. I would get home, find a show to watch (my distraction from reality) and consume every morsel as if it were my last. Ah! Success. I was terribly full, oily and already planning my next meal. Depending on if I was "dieting" or not I would cry in guilt after or wallow in the feeling of being incredibly full. Health articles would suggest cooking more from home. Great idea. Save money and cook for myself proper food portions. What are proper food portions anyway? I would make a box of spaghetti and since there was no one to tell me I shouldn't eat the whole box, I would. If I managed to resist and store left overs in the fridge I would spend the next few hours arguing internally on why I hadn't eaten the left overs yet. Food made me happy so what's the big deal with that? The feeling of happiness would quickly weigh down into depression and guilt and the cycle would continue. The regret of eating so much or eating something "off limits" would become so great I would need to plan my next meal to make me feel better. Let's be honest, I just didn't care. I began to identify with this new-found attitude of I will do what I want. It's my body and I will eat whatever the hell I want! If I want to order a triple meat burger meal and a milkshake at 2 am I should do it! Hell, live a little. Don't even get me started on how alcohol played into my weight gain in college. I am a binge eater! Of course, I was going to be a binge drinker. Drink, its college! These were all the cheerleading moments my addiction and depression used against me to make me feel like I was doing the right thing. Let's be real…treating your body like a punching bag and eating high calorie, sugar filled food into oblivion isn't the right thing to do. It's the easy thing to do.

The inspiring moment to write this book came when I have days I am still not proud of my progress. I'm married, have friends, have a job, hobbies and love my life. Still, those thoughts enter my mind. When I think of children and teens going through what I went through. It's worse now wouldn't you say? Facing your small inner circle as a child in conjunction with the world of social media? Be thin, skinny, tone, tan and happy. I wouldn't trade all the gold in the world to be a child in this decade in time. I was fragile then, I would break under pressure today.

Enough about me. So, you want to change? Tired of feeling like you have no self-control? Maybe just maybe you are some medical anomaly where your brain is wired in such a way that you will never be able to lose weight? I am guessing you live in a cave and have never seen a doctor so that's how you have stayed hidden from the world? Alright, so you're just like me then. Great! Let's be friends. Let's talk about the hardships and the emotional journey weight loss is for people like us. It gets better. Better than I could have ever imagined.

What diets have I tried?

I will name some of the diets that I have tried in my adulthood. I am guessing the strange binge-like diets in my early adulthood don't count. Unless, there is a diet called Eat All the Things, All the Time.

Juice Fasting - drinking fresh pressed juices all day without food
30 Day Juice Cleanse - drinking store bought juices 3x a day for 30 days with no food
5 Day Juice Cleanse – drinking juices to "reboot" my system once a month
Lemon, Cayenne Pepper Drink - you know that nasty stuff people started bottling and selling
If It Fits In Your Macros- eat whatever you want in moderation
Flexible Dieting - eat a strict diet with one "cheat meal"
Whole 30 - eliminating grains, dairy, sugar and eating large portions of meat, veggies and healthy fats
5 – 6 meals a day plan - eating 6 meals a day to eliminate binge eating or hunger
Gym Diet - (Broccoli, Chicken and Sweet potatoes till you die)
Weight Watchers Frozen Meals - eat frozen meals for breakfast, lunch and dinner
Diet Supplements + Meal Plan - diet pills and a cookie cutter meal plan
Vegetarian - no meat
Vegan - no meat, dairy or any animal products
Standard American Diet - (Eat all the things)
The Ketogenic Diet - eliminating grains, sugar and eating high fat, moderate protein, low carb.

Why I chose the Ketogenic Diet?

To be honest, I didn't know too much about the Ketogenic Diet or what all the fuss was about. I decided after a 30-day program on a supplement stack that yet again I had failed. I spent over $200 on a popular and successful supplement stack. It was more of a "bodybuilder" style company and had a huge following of success stories. So yet again, I went all in. I bought the supplements, followed the meal plan and I waited for results. The grand finale? Nothing! Not a single pound. I was going to the gym every day after work. I was choking down pills three times a day and eating what they recommended as healthy. I was spending 3-4 hours on Sunday meal prepping and just getting frustrated. After 30 days, I looked and felt bigger than when I started. I felt stronger but I didn't see any inches off. I was really disappointed. I was convinced that it was me. I have a problem. I MUST have a thyroid, hormone, physiological, astronomical problem! My weight crept up and I took a couple weeks "off" and ate whatever I wanted. You know the drill – give yourself a break and enjoy life. Eat a taco here or there or ten. My husband was a long for the ride. Always game for anything I threw at him. He loves food just as much as I do. But, that isn't his life anymore.

In 2016, he was diagnosed with Crohn's. As much as he and I love food this was a devastating life change. We've struggled with accepting he just can't eat what he once did. So, after my two weeks "off" he started to feel very ill. He is currently on a medication that blocks any symptoms of his disease. So, when he feels ill, we must have really fallen off the wagon. I felt terrible for him, for me, for us. So, I started to look for another solution. I mean at this point I am use to cycling in and out of a diet every 2 months so this was just like any other time.

The Ketogenic Diet came up as a suggestion on my food tracker app. It has a place you can choose a preset meal plan based off of your goals. Every time I entered my stats it would pop up with this "Keto Plan". I kept thinking no I want like a normal "American" plan. I would click all the boxes: need to lose 30 + pounds, lose excessive fat, and lose 2 lbs. per week at an accelerated rate. Enter. The Ketogenic Plan. So, I entertained this stupid app and started researching what it was all about. Breakfast: Eggs, bacon, cream cheese, Lunch: Chicken, broccoli cheese and a side salad, Dinner: Smothered steak, cauliflower mash and salad with full fat dressing. The Keto obsession began. Eat bacon, where do I sign up and let's go buy some damn bacon. This book is NOT to explain the science around the Ketogenic diet and Ketosis. This is for those of us who dove all in and are a bit confused trying to juggle all the books and bacon to make it work.

CHAPTER 2 THE KETOGENIC DIET
NO SCIENCE

The Ketogenic Diet – A high fat, moderate protein, low carb approach to food proportions. If you eat a Standard American Diet (SAD) you are functioning off carbs and sugar. You might think but I don't eat that much sugar. Well, yes you do. How to know if you are carb/sugar fueled? If you eat any one of the following items in a day – you are carb fueled. If you eat 3 or more items in a day you are living the Standard American Diet.

Breakfast includes	Lunch includes	Dinner includes
Oatmeal w/ or w/out sugar, toast, muffins, all cereal, bagels, fruits, biscuits, burritos, pancakes, packaged bars, waffles, doughnuts and any other drink other than black coffee, tea or water	Pasta, sandwiches, wraps, rice dishes, noodle, potatoes, fried foods, pizza, chips, crackers, breaded foods, corn, beans, gravy and salads with 99 croutons and any low-fat foods	Pasta, pizza, fried foods, fried veggies, potatoes, packaged dinner meals, bread, pasta, sandwiches, wraps, rice dishes, noodle dishes, potato heavy, fried foods, pizza, chips, crackers, breaded foods,

Okay so you are carb/sugar fueled. Glad we have that sorted out. Admitting is the first step!

What can your body run off of?
    Carbs - ingested
    Sugar-ingested
    Ketones – produced in the liver
    Fat – stored fat in the body

Facts:

There is only around 1 teaspoon of sugar in our bloodstream needed to survive

Your body produces spikes Glucose and Insulin when you eat ANY foods

Glucose is the chosen fuel if readily available

Insulin is produced to process glucose and escort it around the body

If excess glucose is present, any excess amounts of fat will be stored in your current fat cells

Excess fat that is stored in your fat cells causes your cells to get larger which causes weight gain (the act of expanding each fat cell in your body)

Carbs turn into sugar

Excess protein turns into sugar

The reduction of carbs puts your body into a state of Ketosis

Ketones are produced in the Liver for fuel in the absence of carbs/sugar

For more information on the details of the science behind the Ketogenic Diet indulge in some research and purchase The Ketogenic Bible – newly release with a wealth of information. For now, we will keep it simple.

What we know:

Eat majority healthy fats, moderate protein and little to no carbs. You want your body to run on fat for fuel. Plain and simple. I will explain later which foods are allowed for each macronutrient.

Why Keto works for me?

I have found that my body responds very well to eliminating carbs. How do I know if my body can handle this change? I don't get bloated after eating. I have a serious problem with bloating and I am not talking about gas. When something I eat is carb heavy my intestinal lining will swell like a large hose filling with water. My stomach gets hard, my heart beats fast and I get that drowsy sleepy feeling. I'm like a freaking Anaconda after a Thanksgiving meal. I knew I was sensitive to carbs but I would always attribute it to overeating. In fact, it is my body's response to the flood of glucose, salt and everything else I just ate. So, you might be thinking…what did she eat before Keto? Gallons of ice cream a night? 6 pizzas for dinner? No, I ate a relatively "balanced" American diet with a few cheats. I have had enough practice with dieting that I was able to keep my diet "healthy" for about 4 days out of the week and then I would have a cheat. Monday – Thursday I would be ok and then I would crave pizza, steak, Mexican food and pasta. So, my typical meal plan looked like this:

SAD	B 8 am	L 1 pm	D 6 pm	S 3 pm
M	Hard boiled eggs, deli meat, avocado	Chicken with pasta and sauce	Ground turkey with brown rice and veggies	Nuts
T	Oatmeal w/ brown sugar, fruit and tea	Chicken salad wrap with chips	Turkey salad with dressing and water	String Cheese
W	SKIP	Chicken rice and cheesy veggies	Ground beef, rice and broccoli	String Cheese
TH	Doughnuts at work and juice	Chicken rice and cheesy veggies	Chicken rice and cheesy veggies	
F	Breakfast sandwich with egg and cheese	Chicken with pasta and sauce	½ Pizza hut medium with wings	
S	McDonald's Egg McMuffin and hash brown (rarely)	Mexican food – chips, salsa, enchiladas with rice and beans	Steak, mashed potatoes and zucchini	
SU	SKIP	Chipotle Bowl	Chicken tacos	

As you can see my diet wasn't horrific. I usually ate out on the weekends and during the week those foods were interchangeable. The problem was I was always hungry. I would wake up ready for a full breakfast and then ready for lunch. I was tired when I would get home from work at 6:00 pm. I didn't have the energy to work out and I would drink a gallon of water a day. Most of all, I wasn't losing weight. I was gaining slowly and looking puffy.

Yes, you can be on a no carb diet and lose weight but here is the problem. Hunger. I had a food addiction! Hungry is not in my vocabulary. I cannot tolerate the feeling of being hungry or anything associated with starvation mode. It causes a huge relapse in eating and I will run to the nearest fast food restaurant. I will show you later what my meal plan looks like today and how much my body has changed.

The amazing thing I can actually say is I am not starving. I am not restricting myself in a way that causes obsessive thoughts. I naturally obsess over things so occasionally it happens but not in the cyclical way it used to. It's due to the high amounts of fat in the diet that chemically triggers the feeling of being full (Leptin). It's the same reason I can't drink a milkshake before dinner. Even though it's liquid, the high fat content makes me feel full. Think of fat as a thick layer of paint on your stomach lining. It's heavy, dense and evenly coats the walls giving an overall feeling of fullness. This is the benefit of eating high fat items along with moderate protein and low carb.

CHAPTER 3 I''VE STARTED KETO, NOW WHAT?

Team Keto – Check
Buy full fat cheese – Check
Buy higher fat content meats – Check
Buy low carb veggies – Check
Remove all sugar and carbs from the house – Check
Buy Stevia – Check
Buy an I love Ketosis T- Shirt – Check
Tell everyone in a 30-mile radius that you are KETO ready – Check

Pray to the Keto Gods that you will not eat grains, carb rich veggies, lean meats, low fat cheeses, alcohol or anything that will disrupt K E T O S I S. Ketosis is the Mecca of all that is fat burning. Ketosis is the keeper of all the fat and sends it away out into the universe for ravenous slugs to eat.

So, we are all Keto up in this B****!!! Let's do this.

Wait, what do I do? I'm eating cream cheese on my couch in my Keto Life t-shirt and I'm hungry and not losing weight…HELP!

"Suggested" Daily Macronutrient Guideline Ketogenic Diet
(rough estimate and determined by trial and error)

Carbohydrates - 10%
Protein - 30%
Fat - 60%

The daily amounts I started with
Carbohydrates - 5%
Protein - 15%
Fat - 80%

Let me offer some keto perspective for those who don't track grams or percentages.
Carbohydrates- 5% or 20 grams
Protein – 30% or 58 grams
Fat – 70% or 138 grams
This is what a day would look like

Breakfast	Intermittent Fasting with tea
Lunch: 24g Protein/10g carbs/29g fat	**Roll ups:** 2 slices deli meat with 3 tbs full fat cream cheese, 2 pickle slices and 1 ounce (about 5-6) hazelnuts.
Dinner 34g Protein/13g carbs/79g fat	**Salmon Bowl:** 4 oz. of salmon cooked with 2tbs avocado oil, veggie sauté (2oz mushrooms, ¼ bell pepper, ¼ onion, 2 tbs ghee), 1 poached egg, ½ avocado mixed with 1 tbs organic mayo
Snacks after 3pm	**Moon Cheese or another tea**

So, as you can see by the meal plan I am eating A LOT less than I used to. Honestly, I don't even notice. I still have that syndrome where you pile a bunch of extra food on your plate because you think you can eat it. I can't! My stomach gets full very easily. It's an actual physical feeling now. It's not where I'm mentally telling myself okay now honey, that's enough food. No! It hurts if I eat more than I can. I also get a wave of nausea if I try and push past to eat more. Strange revelation.

Planning

Who loves planning? I do!

I love planning trips, outfits, girl's nights, birthday parties, hair color changes, random DIY projects…but meal planning is no joke!

I recently had my husband try an experiment where he took over the cooking and shopping for one week. He had to choose recipes, make a list, shop and execute all meals. Poor thing. It's a lot for a first timer. I understand those of you who cannot stand the idea of planning out meals and going grocery shopping. Trust me!

Planning will be key on this journey but it won't be forever. Speaking for myself I had to put myself through a cooking boot camp (CBC). It's where I had to basically relearn all my grocery shopping techniques and allowable foods until I had it burned in my mind. If you are willing to give it a try I promise it will be worth it. *whispers* K E T O S I S

P -prepare your meal list (7 lunches, 7 dinners or 14 lunches, 14 dinners)
L- like the food your making (don't make Brussel sprouts and Kale if you want to vomit over it)
A-allow for new things (be open minded to new nuts, flavors and typical dinners)
N-no sugar allowed (this includes sauces and condiments while shopping)

Meal Plans

Meal plans are the most effective way to start and execute a new diet plan. Especially, if you are unfamiliar with where to begin this will be a way to make it work. There are a lot of online meal plans that show a variety of ways to eat on the Ketogenic Diet. WARNING: not all of them will work for weight loss. I have found that some of these preset meal plans are for people that are already Keto Adapted or don't have any excess weight to lose. I like to run through Pinterest or blogs to see what the possibilities are before I default to a preset meal plan.

If you have time to cook dinner look for recipes that require a little more skill and are beautiful to look at. If you work or have kids and dinner can only fit somewhere around 20 minutes total then look for more "lunch style" foods for dinner. Things that you don't have to marinate or spend too much time chopping or peeling will greatly reduce your stress.

Food Diary

The best possible way to calculate the grams of fat, protein and carbs is to track them. There are a variety of apps you can download. I highly suggest if you are first starting out to try and learn to make this a habit. Remember: cooking boot camp (CBC) to make these techniques a habit.

I have found that I can misjudge the amount of protein and carbs greatly if I am not tracking my food.

The great thing about tracking in an app is you can use your preset meal plan to enter all the information ahead of time if you aren't a daily user. The huge benefit is that if you create a meal plan for a day and if you aren't sure if you will hit your numbers, the app will let you know. You can then go back and delete some higher carb or protein items from the list to get those numbers right.

I know a lot of people use MyFitnessPal. I don't blame them! I used MFP for years and years before and it worked great. Frankly, it's a little boring to look at and I needed encouragement. I downloaded the Lifesum app and I have been loving every single day. It has a lot of encouraging tools and even has a preset Ketogenic Diet setting that will change your numbers for you based off of what goals you have. Each meal will show a rating happy face or sad face based off of what you eat. It also tells you how many grams of carbs you went over per meal. How easy is that?

If you decide to download Lifesum find me and add me @jenslyfe. We can be friends and you can look at my entries.

Water

You must drink water. Drink till you are peeing excessively. I use a 73-ounce jug for work and a 32-ounce bottle on the weekends. You can order stylish jugs off Amazon or walk into the Dollar Store and pick one up. The goal for me is to drink 45oz before lunch and then 45 oz. after lunch. Happy peeing!

CHAPTER 4 WHAT HAS PREVENTED MY SUCCESS?

In all diets, you hit those points where you ask yourself "what am I doing wrong?". You're following this preset menu, you're working out or walking, you have cut out sugar, carbs and yet the scale isn't moving. You aren't seeing many changes in your body and it's been weeks. Unfortunately, no one meal plan is right for everyone. We are all made different and we all have different chemistry. I use the term chemistry loosely in that we know from allergies, hormones and caffeine headaches that we are all affected differently. It's no wonder why a plan provided by a 40-year-old male/female who is a marathon runner and isn't looking to lose more weight isn't working for me. No offense to the individual or the meal plan but I need to know what to change about their diet for it to become MY diet. I found more and more with mimicking meal plans that it wasn't right for me. I still needed to lose 30+ pounds, I needed to treat my gut like a porcelain doll she is and I had to stay away from "allowable sugars" at least in the beginning. This is where we start to use our basic body intuition and trial and error.

Too Many Carbs

Nuts on the menu! Awesome. Let's eat all the nuts.

Allowable nuts are:

Macadamia

Almond

Brazil
Walnut
Coconut
Cashew
Hazelnut
Just to name a few

Let me provide some perspective – this could very well be the reason you are not entering Ketosis or losing weight.

Typically, the serving size suggested for nuts is one ounce.
ONE
friggin
OUNCE!

That is the size of what would fit in a golf ball. Reminds me of Easter when you try to fit candy into the Easter eggs. You find that less always makes the egg close easier. In this case, it would be what you can fit into the base of the egg shape. We can't use a generic "handful" approach because in one handful that can be the difference between 160 calories or 400. So, let's take the same list and apply some numbers to them. 1 ounce is a golf ball and a heaping handful is about 2 ounces or 2 golf balls.

Macadamia 2 oz. 467 calories 9g carbs 5g protein 49.3g fat

Almond 2 oz. 410 calories 14g carbs 15g protein 35g fat

Brazil nuts 2oz 401 calories 8.7g carbs 10g protein 47.1g fat

Walnut 2oz 464 calories 9.7g carbs 10.8g protein 46.3g fat

Coconut meat ½ coconut 704 calories 30g carbs 6.6g protein 66g fat

Cashew 2.4oz 390 calories 22g carbs 10.4g protein 31.5g fat

Hazelnut 2.5oz 446 calories 11.9g carbs 10.6g protein 43.2g fat

Well, I know why I didn't enter ketosis when I was munching on mixed nuts twice a day. Truth be told I was on a nut craze. I never use to eat them but essentially, they are a healthy equivalent of chips. So, I kept them in my desk and would eat a few handfuls here and there. My weight loss stopped! Halted! Jumped ship! Limit your nut choices to the ones with less carbs to start out. They are an easy way to boost fat intake but can be stunting if the right ones aren't chosen. You have to start with just one ounce and be strict. Higher fat and less carbs are the way to go. I see you Brazil nut!

Too Much Protein

So, we are on a low carb, high fat diet. Protein is good for you, right? So, let's double up on the chicken at dinner. Get two servings of that delicious bacon at breakfast and eat a whole can of tuna at lunch. Big mistake. Around the same time my weight loss stopped I found myself snacking on salami sticks, jerky, and getting extra servings of meat at dinner. Was I hungry? No, my food addiction was popping up in other forms during my diet. I would sit down to dinner at 6 pm and I would log into my food tracking app to see that I was well over my protein for the day. How could this happen? All I had was chicken at lunch (21g), nuts (24g), steak at dinner (28g) and two servings of cheese (28g). Well, I am no mathematician but my app told me that equals 101g of protein for the day. Remember when I gave you my recommended amounts. 58g of protein was my maximum allotment for the day. That is double! Referencing back to our Keto Facts, excess protein turns into what? Sugar. Just sugar. It was at least a week before I went back through and saw how many days I was over my protein. That did some damage. Tracking is key.

Sneaky "allowable" sugars

No calorie sweeteners are great for making things taste more human like. I don't recommend the use of Stevia daily if you were a soda drinker or chocoholic. It caused me to crave more and more sweet snacks than when I just cut it out completely. I would focus on eliminating it completely and reserve no calorie options for delicious desserts.

Berries

Berries are one of a short list of allowed fruits on Keto. I don't know about you but I love strawberries. I could inhale them and smear them on my face. Blueberries are my next favorite. Midway through my first month I had an intense craving for fruit. It was summer here in Florida and very hot outside. I really wanted a cocktail but I would settle for a dish of strawberries. I ate the whole package. In my mind,

I was like Woo Hoo, Keto, Fat Loss, shake my booty, let's eat some FRUIT. Sigh, that didn't work out too well. I got the same type sugar crash as I would have with a cookie. Limit your allowed berries. I now only use ¼ c of berries for making fat bomb treats. Fat bombs are gold. I will include my favorite recipe in this book.

CHAPTER 5 FOOD ADDICTION & OBSESSION

Overcoming Overeating

Who wants to admit that they overeat till it's physically painful? No one. Can this diet help someone with overeating and obsessive thoughts? Yes. It has for me.

Intermittent Fasting (IF)

After about two weeks on the Ketogenic Diet I wanted to speed up my results just a little bit more. I was starting to develop obsessive thoughts on what to eat for breakfast, lunch and dinner. So, I stumbled upon IF. Basically, you schedule a time in a 24-hour day to fast. I chose to schedule my fasting time after dinner so I can use sleeping to my advantage. I stop eating at 7pm and I will break my fast at noon with lunch. A 17 hour fast for me was what I needed to push me into Ketosis. I stopped craving foods, my energy increased and I have one less meal to buy and plan for. I allow myself to drink water, coffee or tea during my fast. I will typically have water or a hot tea with coconut oil and a dash of creamer in the morning. The added fat first thing in the morning keeps me full and focused for the next few hours. That is when the weight loss started to happen. I highly recommend trying a shorter fast and seeing how long you can extend it. If you wake up hungry, eat. The mornings I wake up ravenous are either because my dinner didn't have enough fat or I exercised too hard the night before.

<u>Falling off the wagon</u>

About two months into my Keto journey I had to travel out of town for my brother's wedding. I was excited and a bit nervous about food choices. I did my research and looked at the hotel menus and found some videos on Keto travel snacks. I was ready. I packed all my snacks, clothes and reading material. I have a video up on my YouTube channel on Keto travel snacks (www.youtube.com/c/jenslyfe).

I was scheduled to be there Tuesday to Friday with the wedding on Thursday. The hotel offered an amazing breakfast buffet and a delicious array of dinners and desserts. Shoot me! My first morning my family invited me to breakfast. I had planned on going to check out the gym instead. I got into gym clothes and walked up the road to breakfast. I told myself just eat eggs and bacon, that's it. Breakfast was a success. Wednesday night we had reservations for the Groom's dinner. An amazing menu of mussels, shrimp cocktail, spinach salads, pork chops, pasta and cheesecakes. Shoot me! I ordered a water, a spinach salad, pork chops with asparagus and potatoes for dinner. All went well until the pork chops arrived in a sweet sea of perfectly mashed potatoes. Mashed potatoes are MY WEAKNESS. Needless to say, I rationalized in that moment that I had been so good thus far that I deserved a treat. I devoured my plate. Poof. Gone. I had one bite of cheesecake to finish off the night and was feeling confident. I was feeling alright until the fullness set in. I was wearing spanx under my dress and that darn thing was obviously cutting off circulation to my stomach. I pulled it down and it was like opening a can of biscuits. My stomach was so swollen and tight I was concerned they would think I smuggled a bath robe inside me. Despair. I felt ashamed. I let mashed potatoes ruin my life in that moment. God they were great though. I forgave myself and woke up the next morning ready to take on the day. Fast forward to lunch time and I was starving. In a strong, intense way that felt all too familiar. I was having a carb/sugar craving like no other. I started to get a headache and salami sticks weren't doing the trick. We went to a little island food hut and ordered something "local". Out came fried chicken wings, seasoned rice and sweet bread. Devoured.

Dinner came and I finished my dinner, coffee and two servings of cake because the 3-year-old next to me didn't eat it. I swear if I look back at photos there must have been the incredible hulk sitting at the table in my place. I felt completely and utterly defeated and awful. I text my husband and told him I did some damage. He ordered some Keto Salts for when I returned to jump back into Ketosis. Things didn't work according to plan on my trip.

In three days, I gained 6 pounds. Sure, I could say it was water weight, travel bloat or it could have been the Chinese food I ate in the Miami airport and the taco bell I ate hours later as a last Hoorah with my husband. All I know is the scale wasn't moving. I tried to flush it out with water, salad, healthy fats, IF, slim tea and exercise. It took me almost 2 weeks to lose the 6 pounds I put on in 3 days. I allowed one cheat as an excuse to go off track and my habit pattern took over and didn't hold back.

If you have a track record like mine I would suggest not tempting yourself for the first few months. Most importantly don't rationalize the reasons why you deserve something off the plan. It's that excuse making that got us into this mess in the first place. Be firm with your goals and take pride in having control at the dinner table. In addition, Miami airport Chinese food sucks. Who knew?

How to use your obsessive tendencies to your advantage?

If you obsess about meals or foods use your mind and manipulate it into craving high fat foods. I created a Pinterest board of Keto foods and saved everything that looked desirable. I would look at the ingredients list and see if everything was Keto approved before saving it.

You could do this for your home or office and save pictures that promote healthy eating. I would change my screensaver on my phone to bacon or avocadoes to remind myself of my plan. If you want to get really crazy Google Keto approved restaurant foods in your area and go nuts.

I truly believe this lifestyle can change your future if you are willing to try. It requires patience, a little bit of research and trial and error. Would you rather spend the next 5 years struggling with weight and being unhappy? I find myself having these moments of "woe is me". I look at people in a restaurant eating what they want, drinking, having dessert and I wonder why can't I have that? I quickly remind myself that I did have all that. I had it all my life and I am miserable. So, let's offer ourselves a deal and promise to be consistent. Consistency is key.

How did my body change?

I have talked a lot about what I have done wrong. Let me share with you some of the amazing things that have happened since I started my Keto journey.

Bloating – I have learned more now than ever that I have a sensitivity to carbs. I had belly bloat aka 9 months pregnant almost every single day of my life. I would get it right after a meal and it would last for hours, sometimes days. It made me feel unhappy, self-conscious and my clothes wouldn't fit. Inflammation can be reduced by eliminating carbs and increasing you water intake. Belly bloating is nonexistent today.

Fatigue – I was a proud endorser of Sloth Life. The life of a sloth is filled with sleep, sleep, naps, food and sleep. My brother and I joke that we were meant to be hibernating bears because we are always down for a good nap or slumber. I can't remember a day when I felt tired. That feeling when 3 pm hits at work and you realize your barely breathing and haven't moved in an hour. I always felt tired, groggy, sinus headache-like and weak. My famous line was "I think I'm getting sick". Can't possibly be my crap diet, I have a real illness. I haven't been sick or even had allergies in months. Just last year I had to drive myself to the Emergency Room because I couldn't breathe. I was told I had an asthmatic attack even though I have never had asthma. They weigh you when you stroll into the ER – I remember being 10 pounds heavier that day and I thought that's why I can't breathe.

Rapid Heart Rate – I am not saying this cures medical conditions or heart arrhythmia. I had my heart checked last year when my health took a bad decline. I wore the heart monitor, ran the stress test and everything was fine. I was just unhealthy and had off the chart levels of Triglycerides. Surprise, Surprise. I don't get heart palpitations anymore and I don't have that hard beating in my chest after walking a short distance. Carry a few bags of groceries around your house and see how hard your body has to work when you put on weight. It can be draining.

Working out – I don't work out nearly as much as I thought I would need to. I use to spend hours in the gym doing random crap that served no purpose. I roughly spend 3 days a week at the most doing light cardio (walking 20-25 minutes), Body weight exercises (20 minutes) or weight training (working arms and legs to keep the skin tight and to build my butt).

Weight loss – I am 5'2 and have an "hourglass" shape (broad shoulders, smaller waist, and wide hips). I lost 20 pounds in my first month and a half on the Ketogenic Diet. I had lost this much weight before but my body composition changed this time around. I have lost close to 20 inches off my body and have seen a huge reduction in cellulite on my legs. My face is thinner and my butt has a shape I recognize (peach emoji). I had over 40% body fat and I still have a lot to lose. I have seen more steady progress than I have ever seen in my life.

Stress – I cannot tell you enough how the stress I felt about meal planning has changed. I dreaded coming up with meal plans on a typical diet because what is considered "healthy" is bland and boring. The ability to cook with butter, oils, fatty meats, cheeses and veggies is culinary freedom. It takes the complication out of dieting and gives you control. I don't have to worry about overeating rice because I don't eat it. I don't have to worry about overeating one bowl of pasta because I don't eat it. I feel freer than before. If I want pizza, I have baked pepperoni with melted cheese and pizza sauce. If I want a quiche, I made a crust less, egg, cheddar and bacon quiche. If I want meat and potatoes, I have smothered pork chops with cheese and onions over garlic, cheddar mashed cauliflower. I was tired of thinking what I couldn't have. I like living by what I can have!

Now that I have you thinking about food. Let's talk about some food!

CHAPTER 6 RECIPES & FATTY THINGS

<u>Top 5 favorite fat filled recipes (dessert & meals)</u>

#1 Blueberry Cheesecake Bites ::squeal::

These are my absolute favorite snacks to have in the freezer whenever I am needing something sweet that isn't chocolate. These are light and perfect to eat on the couch. * Pro tip – you can swap out blueberry for any berry you love.

Ingredients: 4 servings
½ c room temp blueberries (if frozen)
¾ c whipped or regular cream cheese (full fat)
¼ c coconut oil or butter if you prefer
1 tablespoon stevia or 5 drops liquid stevia * sometimes I leave it out
1 tablespoon vanilla extract
1 hand mixer or kitchen top mixer
1 set foil muffin tray or silicone molds (use any shape or size)

1. Make sure the cream cheese, oil and fruit are all at room temperature. If you are using butter make sure you don't microwave it.
2. Wash and dry your blueberries and mash with a fork or blend in a blender.

3. Add the stevia and vanilla to the fruit in a bowl and mix well.
4. Add the cream cheese and oil to the mixture and mix with hand mixer or processor.
5. Give it a taste. If it isn't sweet enough adjust with stevia and vanilla
6. Spoon into your chosen trays and freeze for 1-2 hours or overnight.
7. Enjoy! You can store your remaining fat bombs in a container in the freezer.

Tag me in pictures on Instagram @jenslyfe to show me your bites.

#2 Chicken Bacon Avocado Boats

These are so addictive! A perfect and actually pretty to look at lunch or snack. My husband actually found this recipe and I was shocked at how pretty it was not to mention TASTY.

Ingredients: 2 servings

1 large ripe avocado
1 6-8 oz. grilled chicken breast
2 tablespoons organic mayo or yogurt
1 lime
1 teaspoon of salt
½ bunch of chopped cilantro
1 tablespoon avocado oil
2 cooked crunchy pieces of uncured organic bacon

1. Cook your bacon or buy cooked
2. Crumble up into pieces and split in two for later
3. Grill or bake your chicken breast in avocado oil or bacon grease until cooked
4. Cut your avocado lengthwise and remove pit. Careful not to damage the outer skin (these will serve as your bowls)
5. Scoop out the avocado from each side and mash in a bowl with your mayo, cilantro, salt and lime until smooth. Place bowl to the side

6. Remove your chicken and cut into small cubes. The breast will be divided into two servings.
7. Place the mashed avocado mixture into the two avocado shells evenly.
8. Top with one serving of chicken and one serving of bacon
9. Serve with extra lime if needed
   Enjoy

#3 Bacon & Cheese Smothered Pork Chops w/ Cauli Mash

What can I say about this recipe. Cook it. It is to die for! I don't usually care for pork chops or smothered things but this was exactly what I needed when I had an intense urge for steak and mashed potatoes.

Ingredients: 2 servings

2 bone in pork chops 1 ½ - 2-inch-thick (or two Portobello mushroom steaks to be vegetarian)
1 c shredded cheese – I prefer mozzarella
½ a yellow onion chopped
1 clove garlic minced
1 teaspoon of salt
1 c white button mushrooms
2 slices of crispy cooked bacon
2 tablespoons Bacon grease, ghee or olive oil
2 tablespoons Kerrygold butter
2 tablespoons Dijon mustard
1 package of <u>mashed</u> cauliflower (trader joe's or any other brand) I didn't want to have to boil and mash it myself. The pre-mashed one is very smooth and tasty.

1. Let your pork chops warm to room temperature (10-15 min)
2. Coat both sides of each pork chop with Dijon mustard and salt and set aside
3. Cook your bacon and reserve the grease
4. Melt your butter or ghee in a pan and add your garlic, onion and salt
5. Cook until tender and translucent. Add your mushrooms
6. Cook until mushrooms are soft and remove mixture and set aside
7. Follow the directions of your Mashed Cauliflower and set aside
8. Heat your bacon grease or oil on 4 or Med/low in the same pan
9. Lay your pork chops side by side in your pan and sear for 6-8

min per side depending on the thickness

10. The center of your chops should be firm once each side is seared. You can check by cutting into one or wait till center is firm to the touch
11. Once done turn the stove down to 2 or low and add your cheese divided on each pork chop. Cover with a lid for 2 minutes
12. Now for plating.
13. Divide the mashed cauliflower and place on a plate
14. Remove your chops and place one on each plate
15. Top with mushroom mixture and crumbled bacon
16. Serve and enter Heaven

#4 Crunchy "Tacos" w/ Ground Beef and Quick Guacamole

If you have been missing tacos, crunchy tacos, chips or anything of that nature cheese shells are your new Keto Hero. It sounds more daunting than it actually is. It is best to use a non-stick pan like Gotham pans or Copper Red pans because they don't require the use of butter and just slips out smooth.

You will also need to set aside a stack of napkins to catch the drips of cheesiness.

Ingredients: 2 servings

3 cups shredded cheddar cheese
2 tablespoons Kerrygold butter
½ lb. ground beef
Taco seasoning packet
Green chilies (optional)
1 large avocado
2 tablespoons organic mayo
1/4 bunch of cilantro
1 lime
1 chopped roma tomato
Salt
½ cup of sour cream

1. Make your guacamole however you would like but I keep it simple.
2. Mash avocado and add in chopped tomato, ½ limes juice, ¼ bunch cilantro, salt and 2 tablespoons mayo or yogurt and mash with a fork.
3. Cook your ground beef with the taco seasoning and lime. Start with half the packet and adjust to your liking.
4. Add green chilies if you're feeling adventurous
5. Remove your beef and set to the side
6. In a clean nonstick pan (or greased pan) heat to medium and add 1 ½ c of shredded cheese. Should be a nice single layer of cheese in a circle. Adjust size for the size of the shell you want

7. Heat thoroughly until cheese turns greasy and firm. There should not be a lot of sticky or loose cheese in the center
8. Slide out onto a plate with a napkin and gently fold over with a napkin in between. It will harden in this shape so make it taco like.
9. Repeat for 2 shells or more if you have more cheese
10. Fill your shells with beef and top with sour cream
11. Enjoy with a side of your guacamole

#5 Italian Salmon Bowls

This meal kicks that Italian craving for me pretty quickly. I debated between this one and Zoodles with meatballs. Tough choice but I had to go with this one. Let's challenge ourselves. Why not. I am biased to be honest because I just finished cooking this meal this evening.

Ingredients: 2 servings

1 clove of garlic
1 medium diced onion
1 cup of chopped kale (I buy the ore chopped) or 2 cups of spinach
1 package of basil or 10-12 leaves
4 tablespoons of avocado oil
2 tablespoons of Kerrygold butter
Salt
2 tablespoons of sliced black olives (or half a small can)
1 cup of sugar free marinara sauce or your favorite
1 8oz filet of salmon to split
2 poached eggs (see Google for poaching)

1. Heat 2 tablespoons of avocado oil on medium/low
2. Add your filet and cook 4-5 min a side depending how you like your salmon
3. Once cooked completely remove and set aside. Should be firm
4. Heat the remaining 2 tablespoons of avocado oil and sauté your garlic and onion on medium
5. Cook until translucent and tender and add 2 tablespoons of butter and your shroomies (mushrooms)
6. Cook until tender and add your cup of pasta sauce for 2 min and toss in your basil and kale. Cover with a lid and let simmer on low
7. Poach or fry your eggs to your liking. I love yolk. I am yolk
8. Once the kale is soft and tender you can plate your meal. I like it in a bowl
9. Split the veggie mixture into two bowls and split the salmon

filet equally over both. Add your fancy egg on the side and snap a picture.

Tag me on Instagram because I love food pics! @jenslyfe

CHAPTER 7 FOLLOW MY COOKING VIDEOS

YouTube videos for you! www.youtube.com/c/jenslyfe

I have a small YouTube channel that is mainly for cooking and daily life. Upon release of this book I will be making a Keto series for you to follow. Typically, I show my meal plan, grocery haul and nightly recipes. So, subscribe for frequent updates and please ask questions. Whatever you want to see let me know. I haven't filmed any labeled Keto videos because I wanted to reserve that for the people who purchase this book. You can look back and watch me make meals that are Keto.

Smothered Pork Chops
Breakfast Keto Quiche
Low Carb Lasagna
Keto burgers
Pork Roast Recipe
And plenty others. I hope these recipes make you inspired to get back in the kitchen.

THANK YOU

Thank you for taking a chance on this short book. It's my intent to put out real information about my experiences and journey. It's my hope that you can relate and find solitude in that we are all just trying to figure life out. We can offer guidance and advice to one another to ensure none of us experience hopelessness alone. I am here.

Lifestyle Mastery with Emotional Intelligence:

Master your EQ (Self-Awareness, Self-Management, Social Awareness and Relationship Management)